Homemade Bod
Masks For B

Homemade Body Scrubs And Masks For Beginners

All-Natural Facial Masks & Scrubs To Exfoliate, Nourish, And Induce Healing For Face And Body!

Sarah Brooks

STOP!!! Before you read any further....Would you like to know the secrets of Anti Aging?

If your answer is yes, then you are not alone. Thousands of people are looking for the secret to reducing wrinkles, looking younger, and maintaining a youthful appearance.

If you have been searching for these answers without much luck, you are in the right place!

Not only will you gain incredible insight in this book, but because I want to make sure to give you as much value as possible, right now for a limited time you can get full **100% FREE access to a VIP bonus Ebook** entitled **Anti Aging Made Easy!**

Just Go Here For Free Instant Access:

www.LuxyLifeNaturals.com

Legal Notice

Disclaimer Notice

Table Of Contents

Introduction

I want to thank you and congratulate you for purchasing the book, "Homemade Body Scrubs And Masks For Beginners: 101 Homemade Body Scrubs And Masks for Beginners".

This "Homemade Body Scrubs And Masks For Beginners: 101 Homemade Body Scrubs And Masks for Beginners" book contains proven steps and strategies on how to naturally achieve healthier and more radiant skin with ease. Learn how to give yourself the proper skin care that you deserve by using all-natural ingredients that you can easily find at home!

Each body scrub and mask discussed in this book only takes about five to ten minutes to prepare, and could be applied on the skin in as short as ten minutes. So with fifteen-twenty minutes spent on your skin care regimen every week, you are on your way to achieving more beautiful skin. Caring for your skin has never been this fun and easy!

Thanks again for purchasing this book, I hope you enjoy it!

Chapter 1 - Introduction To Body Scrubs And Masks

The proliferation of facial and body spas all over the country indicates how beauty and wellness have taken the front seat when it comes to good grooming. Interestingly enough, body scrubs and masks are not at all recent innovations, but are actually century-tested rituals that trace their roots back to ancient Egypt and Asia, where natural scrubs and perfume oils were used to moisturize the skin and free it from dirt and wrinkles.

Both facial and body scrubs and masks are meant to exfoliate the skin. Exfoliation is the process of removing dead skin cells so that healthier skin may develop. Exfoliation can be done manually or mechanically, with the use of *scrubs*that are rubbed against the skin, usually with some water in order to remove dead skin. Many house ingredients and materials can be used as a scrub such as sugar and salt crystals, almond shells, sponges and even brushes.

Meanwhile, masks work to exfoliate the skin by creating a natural chemical reaction by which natural ingredients, usually with citric acid and fruit enzymes are applied on the skin and left to dry for some time in order to aid in exfoliation. Fruit juice (like lemon, apple), mud and river clay are some basic items used to create masks. While scrubs are rubbed onto the skin to cause exfoliation, masks are useful for deep-cleansing, healing scars or for whitening skin.

If you think celebrities get all their good looks without exerting any effort, you're wrong. In fact, more and more celebrities are trying to find natural ways to make their skin look naturally beautiful. For instance, Jessica Alba creates her own facial scrub using yoghurt, ground coffee and coconut oil, while Miranda Kerr loves cucumber, and Julia Roberts prefers honey!

While the recipes listed in this book are very easy to make, keep in mind that a good mask or scrub would normally comprise of at least two ingredients. A little tip for beginners is to always store three basic ingredients in the cupboard: sugar, salt and honey. Later, you will understand that most masks and scrubs contain at least one or two of these ingredients.

The next chapters are dedicated to enabling you to come up with different kinds of DIY scrubs and masks that you can apply on your face and on your whole body. Find out which one suits your skin the most, and get ready to have your simple scrub and mask tools that will aid you in achieving that healthy and glowing skin. Go on to Chapter 2!

Chapter 2- Natural Beauty Made Easy

This chapter will discuss some preparations that you will need to make in order to create the most satisfying environment for your beauty ritual. While you may actually survive with just the actual scrub and mask agents on your fingertips, it is best to make your routine more fun and relaxing, so you will be continuously motivated to stick to it.

The Basic Things You'll Need

1. **Mixing bowl.** *This is where you will mix the ingredients for your body scrub and mask.*
2. **Stick brush.** *Although you can use your hands to apply the scrub and the mask on your body, a brush allows you to have the process done more neatly and evenly.*
3. **Gauge spoon.** *This normally comes in 2.5, 5 and 15-ml sizes and helps you make a more accurate mixture for your masks and scrubs.*
4. **Mixing spatula.** *This helps you to evenly mix the ingredients for your mask.*
5. **Exfoliating body cloth.** *Again, you can simply use your hands for your face and body, but an exfoliating cloth will help you finish the process more quickly, and cover areas of your body that may be a bit difficult to reach with your hands.*
6. **Clean towels.** *Make sure that you use different towels for your face and body, since your face tends to be more sensitive. And yes, ensure that these towels are always clean and dry before you use them.*
7. **Moisturizer.** *After a scrub, your skin feels lighter and cleaner, but it also feels more fragile and exposed. A moisturizer will help hydrate your skin and protect it. Products with almond oils and Shea butter work well as moisturizers.*

Remember to dedicate an area in your room or bathroom where

you will do your beauty routine. It is best to do it in a place where water is easily accessible and you can easily relax. If you could put some music on as you go through the routine, then that would be great, too.

While you can apply a body scrub and a body mask while you are seated or standing up, it is best to rest awhile for a couple of minutes after application by lying down. Why do you think body spas are so popular? It's not just the idea of getting better skin, but the whole experience of joy and relaxation that go with it that makes it special.

Chapter 3- Scrub And Mask Basics

Now that you have the tools and equipment for your skin care routine, this chapter will give you an overview of the basic ingredients used in making scrubs and masks for the skin.

All About Ingredients

Several types of scrub and mask ingredients include the following:

1. **Salt-based.** Salt-based body scrubs may be used in different varieties, depending on the grade of sea salt that you want to use for exfoliation. It works best on oily skin. Usually, it is used together with oils– like olive oil, almond oiland sesame oil.
2. **Sugar-based.** A favorite scrub for facials, sugar-based scrubs can make use of either brown or white sugar and is perfect for normal or dry skin. Since it is a bit smoother than salt-based scrubs, it is advisable for those with sensitive skin. Like salt-based scrubs, sugar can also be combined with oils. You can also combine it with honey.
3. **Herbal.** As the name suggests, scrubs and masks can be herbal – cucumber, papaya, strawberry, lemon, apple and avocado are some of the most popular herbal-based masks. In addition, green tea is also fast becoming a popular choice. These are usually combined with essential oils like lavender and chamomile to have a rejuvenating effect on skin, along with a relaxing psychological mindset.

Other ingredients used in scrubs and masks are coffee and milk, but salt, sugar and herbal-based scrubs and masks tend to be more popular. It is good to try different types of scrubs and masks on your skin to get a feel of your own personal preference.

While a scrub is applied by rubbing the mixture on your skin gently with your fingers and having it washed away with tepid water after a couple of minutes, a mask should be left to stay on for a much longer time, normally for about 10-15 minutes. Since both processes aid exfoliation, it is advisable, especially for beginners to choose between a mask and a scrub at one time, instead of using both a mask and a scrub at the same time. A good way to start is to use them alternately every week.

To fully understand the effect of a skin care routine, you must take an effort to **record your progress**. This means that you need to take note of the types of DIY treatments you give your skin and see its visible effects. Write your treatment plan on a notebook or planner, and take pictures of your skin before and after a treatment. This way, you can observe your progress over a period of time and make a valid conclusion on which treatment suits your skin best.

All About Scrubbing

You might think that once you have your mask and scrub, you can just go all out and scrub your body however, you want to, but no. There is a more effective way to apply scrubs, and here are some tips:

1. **Use a body cloth, bath mitt/gloves.** You can reach more parts of your body by using a cloth. In addition, it is also easier to control the pressure of scrubbing when you use one. Remember though – you have to wash them and have them air-dried.
2. **Start from the feet up**. You want to start scrubbing your feet first, in round, circular motions, and then gently go upwards, to scrub the front and back of your legs, torso, arms and neck. The feet are usually the roughest areas to deal with, so you want to handle them first to ensure that they have longer exposure to the scrub's ingredients.
3. **Use a round, circular motion to scrub your skin**. This enables you to rid your body of ingrown hairs, and proves to be gentler than using a back and forth rubbing motion. You can damage your skin if you scrub too roughly, so take your time and scrub gently.
4. **Moisturize**! Remember to hydrate and moisturize your

skin after a good scrub. Take good care of your skin inside and out – drink lots of water and get lots of good skin vitamins by eating walnuts, oat meal, broccoli, low-fat dairy products and even chocolates! Get lots of vitamin C by eating, fruits too!

The Thing About Masks

Masks are easier to use – you just put them on your skin and leave them on for ten-fifteen minutes, after which you rinse them and dry your skin with a towel. Masks are simpler to prepare and normally do not need to have sugar or salt. Most homemade masks contain mud, honey or clay, and are stickier when compared to scrubs. While a mask is easier to use (there are no circular movements to think about or cloths to use), you will normally need to wait a little longer before washing it off.

As a rule of thumb, wait for 10-15 minutes before rinsing off a mask. However, remember that at the first sign of itch or redness, feel free to rinse away as that means you might have extra sensitive skin or have certain allergies that you need to consult with your dermatologist. Oh, and one last thing – never use a mask or scrub on bruised skin.

Now that you are equipped with all of the basics, let's check out some actual recipes you can use. Go to Chapter 4 for your first recipe!

Chapter 4 - Coconut Oil Based Body Scrubs And Mask Recipes

There are two basic advantages to using coconut oil based body scrubs and masks: 1) these are great for softening and moisturizing dry skin and 2) they leave a naturally sweet and delicious smell.

Check out a couple of coconut oil based body scrubs:

1) **Coconut oil and sugar body scrub**. This is the simplest scrub you can use with coconut oil and it is very easy, too.

   a. Mix ¼-1/2 cup of granulated white or brown sugar with ½ cup of coconut oil

   b. Turn on the shower and dampen your skin.

   c. Rub the mixture onto your body using circular motions with your hands and fingers or with a bath cloth. Start with your feet, working upwards to your legs and torso. Make sure that this is done while you are seated, as the oil is slippery and you might fall.

   d. Leave the mixture onto your body for about thirty seconds.

   e. Rinse and pat dry.

   f. Apply your favorite lotion or moisturizer (one with the fragrance of vanilla may do wonders for your sense of smell!)

2) **Vanilla coconut sugar scrub**. Yes! It's almost the same thing but this time you add a secret ingredient: vanilla. You'll need ½ cup of solid coconut oil, a cup of white sugar and some seeds from a vanilla pod. You can vary the

measurements of these ingredients according to your taste.

    a. For this recipe, you can use the same previous method of mixing all three ingredients in a bowl.

    b. For a creamier and fluffier mixture, however, buy solid coconut oil, and whip it for ten minutes.

    c. Add white sugar, along with seeds from a vanilla pod and mix them for about another minute.

    d. Voila! Your vanilla coconut sugar scrub is ready to use. Apply it as usual.

3) **Coconut oil salt scrub**. Want a more vigorous scrub using coconut oil? Try this recipe for some variety – all you need are 2 ½ cups of oil and 1 ½ cups of Epsom salt. Mix the ingredients in a bowl and you're good to go!

4) **Coco-cinnamon scrub.** Mix a cup of brown sugar with half a cup of coconut oil. Add half a teaspoon of cinnamon and an optional teaspoon of vitamin E oil. With this recipe, you'll feel like having a cinnamon dolce latte right after!

Coconut oil works wonders for your skin as a mask, too. Here are some coconut oil recipes for facial masks:

1)   **Coconut-honey mask.** Mix a tablespoon of coconut with 2 teaspoons of honey, and a half teaspoon of lemon juice. Apply the mixture onto your face (make sure to wash your face clean and pat it dry first) and leave on for ten minutes. Rinse with tepid water and pat dry.

2)   **Coco-banana mask.** Having trouble with acne? Make your own coco-banana mask with 1 tbsp. of coconut oil, ½ ripe banana (mashed) and half a teaspoon of turmeric. Combine the ingredients in a bowl and apply it to your skin. Leave it on your skin for 10-15 minutes, wash off and dry.

3) **Coco-mango mask.** Combine a tablespoon of mango pulp and a teaspoon of coconut oil. Mix and use as a mask on your face. Leave it on for 10-15 minutes. If you wish to use it on your whole body, you may do so by adding more ingredients – but you will need a lot of mangoes for sure! This mask can be used for all skin types.

Coconut oil is a very good moisturizing ingredient. It also has a sweet and delicate smell. However, as all the excitement in life comes from variety, be sure to try some other scents and fragrances that may suit your liking. The best way to experiment with fragrances is by using essential oil. Proceed to chapter 5 and get to know the most popular and well-loved essential oils used for taking good care of the skin.

Chapter 5 -Essential Oil Based Body Scrubs And Mask Recipes

"Essential oils" – the very phrase suggests that these oils are quite special, but what are essential oils? An essential oil is a concentrated liquid, normally with aromatic characteristics of the plant where it was extracted from. Essential oils play a major role in aromatherapy. They are also widely used in developing different kinds of fragrances.

When used as a base for scrubs and mask recipes, essential oils tend to be soothing and moisturizing. They are also easily available. There are many essential oils to choose from, but a favorite for making scrubs and masks are the following:

1. **Lavender oil scrub.** So what's the first thing that comes to mind when you hear "lavender"? Rest and relaxation should be on the top of your list! Perfect for aromatherapy and for rejuvenating skin, try this lavender oil scrub recipe: combine ½ cup of Epsom salt or coarse sea salt and 1/3 cup of jojoba oil. Mix these and add 1 tbsp. of dried lavender plus 1 tbsp. of lavender oil. Use the mixture as a scrub. Best used before a good night's sleep.

2. **Lemon oil-coconut body scrub.** This is a scrub best used on your hands – especially if you keep washing dishes and doing the laundry! Mix a cup of white sugar, half a cup of coconut oil and 10-15 drops of lemon essential oil. Use the mixture to scrub your hands – they'll work great on your feet, too!

3. **Rose oil body scrub.** Want a luscious, romantic and sensual body scrub? Try using rose oil as a base ingredient. Use a cup of Epsom salt, 3 tbsps. of rose essential oil, and 3 tbsps. of honey. Mix them all together and use as a scrub/mask. To make your scrub more exciting, crush 6-8 rose petals and add them to the mixture.

4. **Tea tree essential oil scrub.** For oily and acne-prone skin, tea tree oil can do wonders due to its antibacterial properties. Enjoy a light-smelling tea tree oil scrub by doing the following: Make a mixture of 1 cup of sugar, 2 tbsps. of honey and 2 tbsps. of tea tree oil. Use as a scrub/mask on damp skin, rinse and pat off dry.

As you can see, essential oils offer a wide range of options when it comes to making your scrub. Do research on the best brands of essential oils as they tend to make a difference in the effectiveness of the ingredient. In addition, always remember to test the fragrance of the olive oil before putting it into your scrub mixture, as some brands may smell more fragrantly than others, and thus, it will be advisable for you to use only smaller amounts of these types of essential oil so as not to irritate your skin. After all, too much of something won't do your skin any good.

Chapter 6 -Recipes To Exfoliate And Nourish

When it comes to exfoliation and nourishment, nothing beats ingredients like milk, sugar and honey! Exfoliation and nourishment actually go hand in hand when it comes to the skin. The very reason you want to exfoliate is because you want to nourish your skin by removing unwanted, dead skin cells that will allow your healthier skin to show.

Here are some recipes to get your hands on:

1. **Sugar-salt scrub**. Yes! You can have a good time scrubbing your face and body with just two basic ingredients. Get a cup of brown sugar and a half cup of very fine salt. Mix them and use as a scrub! (Don't forget to dampen your skin first, and massage the mixture in a gentle, circular motion. Once done, rinse and pat your skin dry).

2. **Almond-milk body scrub.** Now here's to locking in moisture with milk! Get a cup of finely ground almond meal, ¼ cup of whole milk powder and a cup of bentonite clay for the skin. Add 2 tbsps. of olive oil and use as a scrub. Enjoy!

3. **Milk and sugar scrub/mask.** Now this mix is pretty versatile – you can use it both as a scrub, or leave it on skin for a longer time to use it as a mask. Combine a cup of sugar and 1/3 cup of milk, then add 2 tbsps. of honey and mix. There you go – a sweet facial and body mask is ready!

4. **Banana sugar body scrub.** You won't have to go bananas in order to create your banana sugar body scrub. It's so simple: get a ripe banana, 3 tbsps. of granulated sugar and ¼ tsp. of your favorite essential oil. Mash the banana, mix it with the sugar and add the essential oil and you're good to go. You can use this scrub on both your face

and body, so if you plan to do so, get another banana, along with more sugar and essential oil.

5. **Oat-milk and honey body scrub.** Sure you've heard about oatmeal, but what about oat-milk for a body scrub? Put 1 cup of oatmeal and ½ cup of milk, along with 1/3 cup of honey in your mixing bowl to create this body scrub recipe and have fun! Tip: Leave it on your skin for at least five minutes to maximize the exfoliating effect of oatmeal, and the moisturizing power of milk.

The recipes mentioned in this chapter are especially easy to do as most of the ingredients are easily accessible in your kitchen. Remember to take care of your skin from the inside and out by eating fruits and vegetables, getting enough sleep, engaging yourself in exercise and drinking lots of water. Do this and you're more than halfway to achieving gorgeous-looking skin. However, what happens if you do your scrubs and masks properly once or twice a week as well? Then that means you can say hello to guaranteed radiant skin in as short as two weeks!

Chapter 7 -Coffee Ground Body Scrub And Mask Recipes

Caffeine from coffee can make skin tight and supple. Caffeine is known for its ability to reduce the appearance of cellulites. It smoothens skin and makes a very good exfoliant. You can apply coffee topically under eye bags to reduce dark circles. Nevertheless, coffee makes a very good body scrub ingredient.

1. **Coffee-coconut scrub**. Combine a cup of ground coffee with 3 tbsp. of coconut oil, 1 tbsp. of essential oil (ginger will work perfectly) and 1 cup of sugar. You can also add moisturizing oil like jojoba. Use it as a body scrub. Rinse well and pat dry.

2. **Coffee-vanilla sugar scrub**. Make a mixture of ½ cup ground coffee, 1 ½ cup of sugar, 2 tsp. vanilla extract and ½ cup of jojoba oil. You can add 1-2 tsp. of vitamin E oil and essential oil to make this scrub more hydrating.

3. **Coffee-honey mask.** Make a very quick and simple mask by using 1 tbsp. of ground coffee and 1 tsp. of honey. This is simple and easy to do, but it's quite effective as the honey moisturizes your skin and the coffee exfoliates it well.

4. **Coffee-egg mask.** This literally bittersweet mask works very well in exfoliating your face. Mix 1 tbsp. of used coffee grounds with 1 tsp. of sugar, 1 egg and 1 tbsp. of honey. Apply the mixture onto your face and leave for ten-fifteen minutes. Rinse off with cold water and dry.

5. **Coffee-cocoa facial mask.** Talk about antioxidant power with these two brown powders! Combine 3 tbsps. of unsweetened cocoa powder, 3 tbsps. of ground coffee beans and 8 tbsps. of unflavored yogurt. Use the mixture as a mask. Note that you can modify this mask by adding 1-2 tbsps. of lemon juice or lemon essential oil if you want to

have a more brightening effect. Meanwhile, you can also add honey if you have extra dry skin.

It is amazing how coffee can turn out not only to be your favorite drink, but also your most loved skin care product! Coffee masks and scrubs tend to be stimulating and invigorating; indeed, it somehow offers the same experience when you drink your coffee. Your skin will look youthful, full of life and energy!

Chapter 8 - Avocado Mask Recipes

Like carrots, avocados are good for the skin because they are high in antioxidants and vitamins C and E. Using avocado can help fight free radicals in the skin and aid in the regeneration of skin cells. Avocado can function as some sort of sunscreen, and at the same time, reduces and prevents the appearance of breakouts and wrinkles.

Nourish your skin with an avocado mask by trying out these versatile avocado recipes:

1. **Avocado-lemon mask.** Mash an avocado to make ½ cup and mix it with 1 egg white and a teaspoon of freshly squeezed lemon juice; use the mixture as a mask to leave on for 15 minutes. This will rid your skin of excess oil and help you achieve a lighter complexion.

2. **Avocado-honey mask.** Want a simple avocado recipe for your dry skin? Mash 2 tbsps. of avocado and mix it with a tbsp. of honey. Apply onto your face and leave on as a mask for 10-15 minutes, rinse and pat dry. Once done, don't forget to put on some moisturizer!

3. **Avocado-sugar mask**. Say you don't have honey, but have avocado. You can still make a good mask out of that for your skin! Mash half an avocado and mix it with 1 tbsp. of sugar. Add 1-2 tbsps. of olive oil and try it on your face.

4. **Avocado-milk mask.** For softer skin with a smoother feel, try this avocado milk mask: Make a mixture consisting of half a cup of mashed avocado, 1/3 cup of honey and 1/3 cup of milk. Add some sugar for better exfoliation and use as a mask.

5. **Avocado-strawberry mask.** Want clean and well-toned skin? Try this vitamin-packed avocado-strawberry mask:mash two-three strawberries and ½ of an avocado,

along with 2 tbsps. of honey and 2 tbsps. of coconut oil. Slather the mixture on your face and rinse after ten-fifteen minutes.

Whether or not avocado is your favorite fruit, there is no doubt that it is one of the best fruit skin care items you'll ever find, and one of the easiest fruits to use in making scrubs, too. It can be easily mashed, and makes a fitting mask, don't you think?

Chapter 9 - Cucumber Mask Recipes

Best known in the beauty industry for its ability to reduce dark circles under the eyes, cucumbers make wonderful and relaxing masks. Cucumber is best used for skin rejuvenation and revitalization. It can be used to lessen the appearance of freckles and blemishes. It can brighten skin, soothe sunburn and reduce the appearance of cellulites.

Making a cucumber mask is relatively easy. Here are some cucumber mask recipes you can try at home:

1. **Cucumber-yogurt mask.** Start very simply with a cucumber-yogurt mask that fits all skin types. Peel ½ cucumber and mix it with 1 tbsp. of unflavored yogurt. You can add a tbsp. of honey if you have dry skin. Use as a mask and leave it on for 10-15 minutes and rinse off with tepid water.

2. **Sugary-cucumber mask.** Peel and blend 1/2 cucumber into a puree and combine it with half a cup of brown sugar and 2 tbsps. of honey. Add an optional 1/3 cup of milk for extra moisture.

3. **Cucumber-egg mask.** Why add an egg to your cucumber mask? That's because a protein-rich egg can help you achieve tighter, younger-looking skin and minimize the appearance of your pores. Start by pureeing half a cucumber as usual, mix it with 1 egg (remove the yolk) and 1/3 cup of brown sugar.

4. **Cucumber-milk mask.** For a clean and moisturizing feel, try having a cucumber-milk mask. Puree half of a small cucumber and put it in a mixture of milk (1/4 cup), honey (2 tbsps.) and sugar (2 tbsps.). It can be tempting to turn the whole thing into a drink, but it's really good for your skin!

5. **Cucumber-oatmeal mask.** Here's a cool, exfoliating mask recipe: Puree ½ cucumber and combine it with 1 tsp. of honey, 1 tbsp. of oatmeal and 4-5 drops of peppermint essential oil. Use the mixture as a mask and leave on for 10 minutes. Rinse off, dry and use a moisturizer.

As you enjoy wearing a cucumber mask when relaxing and waiting for that magical ten or fifteen minutes, maximize your time by making two slices of cucumber that you can put on your eyes. You've seen it in the movies, why don't you try it, too?

Chapter 10 - Carrot Mask Recipes

Carrots are rich in antioxidants and have vitamin A and vitamin C, making them a real skin care booster whether eaten or applied on skin. When used as a scrub or a mask, carrots can tone and lighten skin, giving it a beautiful, lively and bright color. Carrots can also help repair skin damage and rid the skin of free radicals. It is one of the base ingredients of masks that is generally appropriate for all skin types.

Here are some DIY carrot mask recipes:

1. **Carrot-lemon mask.** Peel half a carrot, boil it and then mash it. Once it has cooled, mix it with 1 tsp. of freshly squeezed lemon juice. Add 2 tbsps. of honey. Use this facial mask to have clean and well-toned skin that is suitable for all skin types.

2. **Carrot-honey face mask.** Peel the skin off 1 small carrot, boil and mash until creamy. Add 2 tbsps. of honey and 2 tbsps. of water. You can also add some brown sugar (1 tbsp.) to this mixture, along with some olive oil (1 tbsp.) to help smoothen your dry skin.

3. **Carrot-avocado mask.** Remember all the skin benefits of avocado? Pair it with a carrot and enjoy a deeply moisturizing mask that can soften usual problem areas like the knees and elbows. Here's the recipe: Peel 1 avocado and 1 carrot. Grate the carrot and mash the avocado, add 1 tbsp. of Epsom salt along with 2 tbsps. of olive oil. Apply onto skin and leave on for 10-15 minutes.

4. **Carrot-sugar scrub.** Have no time to boil those carrots? Grate half a carrot after you peel them, put 2 tbsps. of sugar and 2 tbsps. of honey. Stir it well and you'll have a good homemade version of a carrot scrub without the hassle of having to "cook" the carrot.

5. **Carrot-coconut mask.** Want well-toned skin without breakouts? Use this simple carrot-coconut mask recipe: Boil 1 small carrot, mash it and leave it to cool. Add 1-2 tbsps. of coconut oil and mix. Apply the mask to your face and leave it for 5-10 minutes. Rinse and pat dry.

The carrot might as well be the best natural toner you can ever get! It may take some time in terms of preparation, as you usually need to boil it in water before you mash it, but this is definitely worthwhile. Try to give yourself a carrot-based mask at least once a month.

There may be many other recipes out there to choose from, so continue to read about new trends in facial care in various magazines and beauty websites. As you enjoy trying out a new recipe every week or every month, do not forget to record the types of masks or scrubs that you feel work best on your skin. Each person has a different kind of requirement when it comes to skin care, so there is really no such thing as a one size fits all skin care regimen.

Conclusion

Thank you again for purchasing this book on *Homemade Body Scrubs And Masks For Beginners: 101 Homemade Body Scrubs And Masks For Beginners!*

I am extremely excited to pass this information along to you, and I am so happy that you now have read and can hopefully implement these strategies going forward.

I hope this book was able to help you understand skin care in a better light and learn how to prepare your own natural and homemade body scrubs and masks.

The next step is to get started using this information and to hopefully live a more beautiful and exciting life – even when it comes to the simple joy of caring for your skin!

Please don't be someone who just reads this information and doesn't apply it, the strategies in this book will only benefit you if you use them!

If you know of anyone else that could benefit from the information presented here please inform them of this book.

Finally, if you enjoyed this book and feel it has added value to your life in any way, please take the time to share your thoughts and post a review on Amazon. It'd be greatly appreciated!

Thank you and good luck!

Preview Of:

Anti Inflammatory Diet: The #1 Anti Inflammatory Recipe Guide!

<u>Anti Inflammatory Diet</u>

Eliminate Pain, Heal Yourself, Combat Heart Disease, And Fight Inflammation Using Food!

Introduction

I want to thank you and congratulate you for purchasing the book, *"Anti Inflammatory Diet: Anti Inflammatory Diet: The #1 Anti-Inflammatory Recipe Guide! - Eliminate Pain, Heal Yourself, Combat Heart Disease And Fight Inflammation Using Food"*.

This "Anti Inflammatory Diet" book contains proven steps and strategies on how to fight inflammation through holistic approach.

Inflammation is the body's natural response to infection and injuries. It is essential to start the healing process. Redness, pain, swelling and heat are symptoms which mean that the body is triggering the immune system to fight foreign bodies and start tissue repair. The problem arises when the healthy cells are damaged in the aftermath of inflammation.

Inflammation is linked to major chronic illness like heart diseases, stroke and diabetes. Fortunately, people are not powerless in preventing inflammation from going out of control. By ensuring that you have a healthy lifestyle, you are relieving your body from toxins and prevent common chronic illness.

Adopting healthy habits can dramatically improve your inflammation symptoms. This is a combination of a healthy diet and good habits. Fuel your body with natural anti-inflammatory foods to keep your joints functioning well.

Take control of your life and start living a healthy lifestyle to feel better.

Thanks again for purchasing this book, I hope you enjoy it!

Chapter 1: Anti-inflammatory Diet Guidelines

Unlike other diets, the anti-inflammatory diet is different since it is solely focused on weight loss. It is more of a dietary guideline for life than a short term diet.

There are also more than one approach to the anti-inflammatory diet with each one having its own benefit. Many doctors say that the anti-inflammatory diet can benefit everyone and is good for overall health.

What is inflammation?

Inflammation is the body's response to harmful and irritating stimuli. It is the body's way of protecting itself by removing damaged cells, pathogens and irritants to encourage a faster healing process.

Inflammation is not the same as infection although infection can cause inflammation. Infection is caused by virus, fungus and bacteria while inflammation is the body's reaction to it.

Initially, inflammation is beneficial to your immune response. For example, if you cut yourself while cooking, you might notice the area swells and reddens. This response is essential in the healing process.

Types of inflammation

- Acute inflammation

Acute inflammation starts rapidly as soon as the injury is acquired. It can last for few minutes to only few days. The most common examples of acute inflammation are cuts, bruises and sore throat.

- Chronic inflammation

Chronic inflammation is long term and can even last for years. It usually results after the body has failed to eliminate the cause of acute inflammation. It is also a response to antigens. It happens when the body attacks healthy tissue because it mistakes it for harmful pathogens. Examples include asthma, tuberculosis and chronic sinusitis.

Signs of inflammation

- Pain. The inflicted area will be painful most especially when touched. Chemicals in the body are released in the nerve ending making the area much more sensitive.
- Redness. The redness happens because the capillaries are filled with more blood than usual.
- Immobility. Since the area is painful to touch, you might also experience loss of function.
- Swelling. This is caused by the accumulation of fluid in the affected area.
- Heat. More blood accumulates in the area which makes it warmer than the rest of the body.

What happens during inflammation?

You can feel the effect of inflammation immediately after the tissue is damaged. Acute inflammation occurs in three stages. First, the arterioles or the small branches of the arteries that supply blood to the different parts of the body dilate and results to an increase in blood flow. The capillaries become permeable and fluid and blood move in-between the spaces of cells. Neutrophilis which is a type of white blood cell that contains enzyme that digest microorganisms move out of the capillaries. It then transfers to the spaces between the cells.

The Neutrophilis is the body's first line of defense since it contains enzymes that can destroy bacteria and prevent infections. However, it also contains inflammatory properties which can lead to heart ailments and autoimmune disease.

Function of the anti-inflammatory diet

Physicians and medical experts may recommend anti-inflammatory diets to lessen the effect of inflammation in the body. The diet is usually prescribed with other medicines but you can also follow it to simply reduce inflammation symptoms in your system. Adding foods that improve symptoms of chronic disease supplies the body with the needed nutrients to decrease body inflammation.

Thanks for Previewing My Exciting Book Entitled:

"Anti-Inflammatory Diet: The #1 Anti Inflammatory Recipe Guide! Eliminate Pain, Heal Yourself, Combat Heart Disease, And Fight Inflammation Using Food!"

To purchase this book, simply go to the Amazon Kindle store and simply search:

"ANTI-INFLAMMATORY DIET"

Then just scroll down until you see my book. You will know it is mine because you will see my name "Sarah Brooks" underneath the title.

Alternatively, you can visit my author page on Amazon to see this book and other work I have done. Thanks so much, and please don't forget your free bonuses

DON'T LEAVE YET! - CHECK OUT YOUR FREE BONUSES BELOW!

Free Bonus Offer: Get Free Access To The www.LuxyLifeNaturals.com VIP Newsletter!

Once you enter your email address you will immediately get free access to this awesome newsletter!

But wait, right now if you join now for free you will also get free access the "Secrets of Becoming A Meditation Expert – In 7 Days!" free Ebook!

To claim both your FREE VIP NEWSLETTER MEMBERSHIP and your FREE BONUS Ebook on the SECRETS OF BECOMING A MEDITATION EXPERT IN 7 DAYS!

Just Go To:

www.LuxyLifeNaturals.com

CPSIA information can be obtained
at www.ICGtesting.com
Printed in the USA
LVOW10s0858131116

512778LV00027B/518/P

9 781519 345639